The Zero Stress Zero Points Weight Loss Cookbook

Delicious No-Point Recipes for Fast Weight Loss, Improved Health, and Easy Meal Planning

Dr. Myles Watson Collins

Copyright © 2024 by Dr. Myles Watson Collins

About the Author

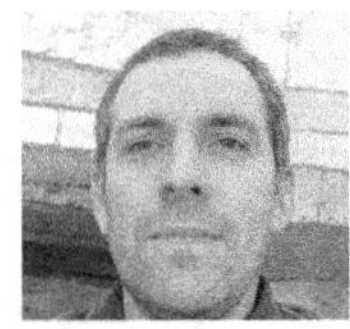 Dr. Myles Watson Collins is a respected nutritionist and wellness expert with over 20 years of experience in the field. He holds a Ph.D. in Nutrition Science and has dedicated his career to helping individuals achieve their health and wellness goals through practical, evidence-based strategies. Dr. Collins is a passionate advocate for healthy eating and believes that nutritious food should be both delicious and accessible to everyone. He has authored several books and articles on nutrition and regularly speaks at health and wellness conferences and workshops. Dr. Collins is committed to empowering people to live healthier, happier lives through better food choices and lifestyle habits.

Dear Readers,

If you enjoyed reading and using this book, please leave a review. Your feedback means a lot to me and helps others discover the book. I will really appreciate it.

Thank you!

Contents

Introduction

Welcome to the world of no-point cooking, where you can enjoy delicious meals without the stress of counting points or calories. This book, "The Zero Stress Zero Points Weight Loss Cookbook: Delicious No-Point Recipes for Fast Weight Loss, Improved Health, and Easy Meal Planning," is designed to help you achieve your weight loss goals and improve your health through easy, tasty, and healthy recipes. Whether you're a seasoned cook or just starting out in the kitchen, this guide will provide you with everything you need to succeed on your no-point journey.

Understanding the No-Point System

The no-point system is a simple and effective way to manage your diet without the hassle of tracking every bite you eat. Instead of assigning point values to foods, this system focuses on naturally low-calorie, nutrient-dense foods that you can enjoy freely. These include fruits, vegetables, lean proteins, and whole grains. By building your meals around these no-point foods, you can eat until you're satisfied without worrying about exceeding your daily points allowance.

The beauty of the no-point system lies in its simplicity. There are no complicated calculations or rigid rules to follow. Instead, you have the freedom to create meals that fit your tastes and lifestyle while still supporting your weight loss and health goals. This approach encourages mindful eating and helps you develop a healthy relationship with food.

Benefits of No-Point Recipes

No-point recipes offer numerous benefits that make them an excellent choice for anyone looking to lose weight and improve their health. Here are some key advantages:

1. **Simplicity**: No-point recipes are easy to follow and don't require detailed

tracking. This makes meal planning and preparation straightforward and stress-free.

2. **Flexibility**: With no-point recipes, you have the freedom to choose from a wide variety of foods. This flexibility allows you to enjoy a diverse and satisfying diet.

3. **Nutrient-Dense**: No-point foods are naturally rich in essential nutrients, vitamins, and minerals. This means you can nourish your body while still working towards your weight loss goals.

4. **Sustainability**: The no-point system promotes a balanced and sustainable approach to eating. It's not about restrictive dieting but about making healthier choices that you can maintain in the long run.

5. **Satiety**: By focusing on whole, unprocessed foods, no-point recipes help you feel full and satisfied. This can reduce the temptation to overeat or indulge in unhealthy snacks.

How to Use This Cookbook

This cookbook is designed to be your go-to resource for no-point cooking. Each chapter is filled with delicious recipes that are easy to prepare and fit perfectly into your no-point lifestyle. Here's how to make the most of this book:

1. **Start with the Basics**: Begin by familiarizing yourself with the no-point system and the benefits of no-point recipes. This will give you a solid foundation for your journey.
2. **Explore the Chapters**: Each chapter focuses on a different meal type, from breakfasts and lunches to dinners, snacks, and desserts. Browse through the recipes and choose the ones that appeal to you.
3. **Follow the Recipes**: Each recipe includes simple, step-by-step instructions to guide you through the cooking process. Don't be afraid to experiment and make adjustments to suit your taste.

4. **Use the Food Lists**: This cookbook provides comprehensive no-point food lists and pantry staples. Use these lists to stock your kitchen with essential ingredients.

5. **Stay Motivated**: The final chapter offers tips and encouragement to help you stay motivated on your no-point journey. Remember, the goal is to enjoy the process and make lasting changes to your eating habits.

Essential Kitchen Tools for No-Point Cooking

To make your no-point cooking experience as smooth and enjoyable as possible, it's helpful to have a few essential kitchen tools on hand. Here are some items that will come in handy:

1. **Good Quality Knives**: A sharp chef's knife and a paring knife are essential for chopping and preparing ingredients.

2. **Cutting Boards**: Have separate cutting boards for vegetables, fruits, and proteins to prevent cross-contamination.
3. **Measuring Cups and Spoons**: Accurate measurements are key to following recipes correctly.
4. **Mixing Bowls**: A set of mixing bowls in various sizes will help you mix, toss, and prepare ingredients.
5. **Non-Stick Cookware**: Non-stick pans and pots make cooking and cleanup easier.
6. **Blender or Food Processor**: Useful for making smoothies, sauces, and purees.
7. **Baking Sheets and Pans**: Essential for baking no-point snacks and desserts.
8. **Storage Containers**: Keep your no-point meals fresh with airtight containers.

Having these tools in your kitchen will make no-point cooking more efficient and enjoyable. As you begin to explore the recipes in this book, you'll find that preparing healthy, delicious meals can be both easy and fun.

In the following chapters, you'll discover a wide range of no-point recipes designed to help you lose weight, improve your health, and enjoy every bite. So, let's get started on this exciting journey to a healthier, happier you!

Chapter 1: Energizing Breakfasts

Starting your day with a nutritious, no-point breakfast sets the tone for healthy eating throughout the day. Energizing breakfasts give you the boost you need, keeping you full and satisfied until your next meal. In this chapter, you'll find a variety of breakfast options that are quick to prepare, high in protein, and packed with flavor. Let's dive into some delicious no-point breakfast ideas!

1.1 Quick and Easy Breakfast Ideas

Mornings can be hectic, but that doesn't mean you have to skip breakfast or settle for unhealthy options. Here are some quick and easy no-point breakfast ideas that you can whip up in minutes:

1.1.1 Avocado Toast with Tomato and Basil

- **Prep Time:** 5 minutes
- **Cook Time:** 2 minutes
- **Servings:** 1
- **Ingredients:**
    1. 1 slice of whole-grain bread
    2. 1/2 ripe avocado, mashed
    3. 1 small tomato, sliced
    4. Fresh basil leaves
    5. Salt and pepper to taste
- **Instructions:**
    1. Toast the bread until golden brown.
    2. Spread the mashed avocado on the toast.
    3. Top with tomato slices and basil leaves.
    4. Season with salt and pepper.

1.1.2 Greek Yogurt with Berries

- **Prep Time:** 3 minutes
- **Cook Time:** 0 minutes
- **Servings:** 1

- **Ingredients:**
    1. 1 cup of non-fat Greek yogurt
    2. 1/2 cup of mixed berries (strawberries, blueberries, raspberries)
    3. 1 tablespoon of chia seeds
- **Instructions:**
    1. Place the Greek yogurt in a bowl.
    2. Top with mixed berries and chia seeds.
    3. Enjoy immediately.

1.1.3 Veggie Omelette

- **Prep Time:** 5 minutes
- **Cook Time:** 5 minutes
- **Servings:** 1
- **Ingredients:**
    1. 3 egg whites
    2. 1/2 cup of chopped spinach
    3. 1/4 cup of diced bell peppers
    4. 1/4 cup of sliced mushrooms
    5. Salt and pepper to taste
- **Instructions:**

1. Heat a non-stick skillet over medium heat.
2. Add the bell peppers and mushrooms, cooking until softened (about 3 minutes).
3. Add the spinach and cook until wilted (about 1 minute).
4. Pour the egg whites over the veggies and cook until set (about 2 minutes).
5. Season with salt and pepper.

1.2 High-Protein Breakfasts for a Great Start

Protein is essential for a filling breakfast that keeps you energized throughout the morning. These high-protein, no-point breakfast recipes are both delicious and satisfying:

1.2.1 Scrambled Eggs with Spinach and Feta

- **Prep Time:** 5 minutes
- **Cook Time:** 5 minutes

- **Servings:** 1
- **Ingredients:**
    1. 2 whole eggs and 2 egg whites
    2. 1/2 cup of fresh spinach, chopped
    3. 1/4 cup of crumbled feta cheese
    4. Salt and pepper to taste
- **Instructions:**
    1. In a bowl, whisk together the eggs and egg whites.
    2. Heat a non-stick skillet over medium heat.
    3. Add the spinach and cook until wilted (about 1 minute).
    4. Pour the egg mixture into the skillet and cook, stirring frequently, until the eggs are scrambled (about 3 minutes).
    5. Sprinkle with feta cheese and season with salt and pepper.

1.2.2 Cottage Cheese and Fruit Bowl

- **Prep Time:** 3 minutes
- **Cook Time:** 0 minutes
- **Servings:** 1

- **Ingredients:**
    1. 1 cup of low-fat cottage cheese
    2. 1/2 cup of sliced peaches or any other fruit
    3. 1 tablespoon of honey (optional)
- **Instructions:**
    1. Place the cottage cheese in a bowl.
    2. Top with sliced peaches or your fruit of choice.
    3. Drizzle with honey if desired.

1.2.3 Protein Pancakes

- **Prep Time:** 5 minutes
- **Cook Time:** 10 minutes
- **Servings:** 2
- **Ingredients:**
    1. 1 ripe banana
    2. 2 eggs
    3. 1/2 teaspoon of baking powder
    4. 1/4 cup of rolled oats
    5. 1/4 cup of non-fat Greek yogurt
    6. Fresh berries for topping
- **Instructions:**

1. In a blender, combine the banana, eggs, baking powder, oats, and Greek yogurt. Blend until smooth.
2. Heat a non-stick skillet over medium heat.
3. Pour the batter onto the skillet to form pancakes.
4. Cook for 2-3 minutes on each side, until golden brown.
5. Top with fresh berries and serve.

1.3 No-Point Smoothies and Juices

Smoothies and juices are a great way to pack in nutrients quickly and easily. Here are some no-point options to get you started:

1.3.1 Green Detox Smoothie

- **Prep Time:** 5 minutes
- **Cook Time:** 0 minutes
- **Servings:** 1
- **Ingredients:**
    1. 1 cup of spinach

2. 1/2 cucumber, chopped
3. 1 green apple, cored and chopped
4. 1/2 lemon, juiced
5. 1 cup of water

- **Instructions:**
    1. Place all ingredients in a blender.
    2. Blend until smooth.
    3. Pour into a glass and enjoy immediately.

1.3.2 Berry Blast Smoothie

- **Prep Time:** 5 minutes
- **Cook Time:** 0 minutes
- **Servings:** 1
- **Ingredients:**
    1. 1 cup of mixed berries (strawberries, blueberries, raspberries)
    2. 1/2 banana
    3. 1 cup of unsweetened almond milk
    4. 1 tablespoon of chia seeds
- **Instructions:**

1. Place all ingredients in a blender.
2. Blend until smooth.
3. Pour into a glass and enjoy immediately.

1.3.3 Tropical Delight Smoothie

- **Prep Time:** 5 minutes
- **Cook Time:** 0 minutes
- **Servings:** 1
- **Ingredients:**
    1. 1 cup of pineapple chunks
    2. 1/2 mango, peeled and chopped
    3. 1/2 banana
    4. 1 cup of coconut water
- **Instructions:**
    1. Place all ingredients in a blender.
    2. Blend until smooth.
    3. Pour into a glass and enjoy immediately.

1.4 Overnight Oats and Breakfast Bowls

Overnight oats and breakfast bowls are perfect for busy mornings when you need a grab-and-go option. Here are some delicious no-point recipes:

1.4.1 Classic Overnight Oats

- **Prep Time:** 5 minutes (plus overnight)
- **Cook Time:** 0 minutes
- **Servings:** 1
- **Ingredients:**
    1. 1/2 cup of rolled oats
    2. 1/2 cup of unsweetened almond milk
    3. 1/2 banana, sliced
    4. 1/4 cup of blueberries
    5. 1 tablespoon of chia seeds
- **Instructions:**
    1. In a jar or bowl, combine the oats, almond milk, banana, blueberries, and chia seeds.
    2. Stir well and cover.
    3. Refrigerate overnight.
    4. In the morning, give it a stir and enjoy.

1.4.2 Peanut Butter Banana Overnight Oats

- **Prep Time:** 5 minutes (plus overnight)
- **Cook Time:** 0 minutes
- **Servings:** 1
- **Ingredients:**
    1. 1/2 cup of rolled oats
    2. 1/2 cup of unsweetened almond milk
    3. 1 tablespoon of natural peanut butter
    4. 1/2 banana, sliced
    5. 1 tablespoon of flax seeds
- **Instructions:**
    1. In a jar or bowl, combine the oats, almond milk, peanut butter, banana, and flax seeds.
    2. Stir well and cover.
    3. Refrigerate overnight.
    4. In the morning, give it a stir and enjoy.

1.4.3 Acai Breakfast Bowl

- **Prep Time:** 10 minutes
- **Cook Time:** 0 minutes
- **Servings:** 1
- **Ingredients:**
    1. 1 packet of frozen acai puree
    2. 1/2 banana
    3. 1/2 cup of mixed berries
    4. 1/4 cup of granola (optional, check for no added sugars)
    5. 1 tablespoon of coconut flakes
- **Instructions:**
    1. In a blender, combine the acai puree, banana, and mixed berries. Blend until smooth.
    2. Pour the mixture into a bowl.
    3. Top with granola and coconut flakes.
    4. Enjoy immediately.

These breakfast recipes will help you start your day on the right foot, providing the energy and nutrients you need without any stress. Enjoy these no-point options and feel great knowing you're fueling your body with healthy, delicious foods!

Chapter 2: Satisfying Lunches

Lunch is a crucial meal that keeps you fueled through the afternoon. With these no-point recipes, you can enjoy a variety of satisfying and nutritious lunches without worrying about counting points. From fresh salads and hearty soups to light wraps and meal prep tips, this chapter has everything you need to create delicious and healthy lunches.

2.1 No-Point Salads and Dressings

Salads are a fantastic way to pack in a variety of nutrients while keeping your meals light and refreshing. Here are some no-point salads and dressings to keep you satisfied:

2.1.1 Mediterranean Chickpea Salad

- **Prep Time:** 10 minutes
- **Cook Time:** 0 minutes
- **Servings:** 2
- **Ingredients:**
    1. 1 can of chickpeas, drained and rinsed
    2. 1 cup of cherry tomatoes, halved
    3. 1 cucumber, diced
    4. 1/4 red onion, thinly sliced
    5. 1/4 cup of Kalamata olives, pitted and halved
    6. 1/4 cup of crumbled feta cheese
    7. Juice of 1 lemon
    8. 2 tablespoons of extra-virgin olive oil
    9. Salt and pepper to taste
    10. Fresh parsley, chopped
- **Instructions:**
    1. In a large bowl, combine the chickpeas, cherry tomatoes, cucumber, red onion, and olives.

2. Add the feta cheese, lemon juice, olive oil, salt, and pepper. Toss to combine.
3. Garnish with fresh parsley and serve immediately.

2.1.2 Asian Cabbage Salad

- **Prep Time:** 15 minutes
- **Cook Time:** 0 minutes
- **Servings:** 2
- **Ingredients:**
    1. 2 cups of shredded green cabbage
    2. 1 cup of shredded purple cabbage
    3. 1 carrot, julienned
    4. 1 red bell pepper, thinly sliced
    5. 2 green onions, chopped
    6. 1/4 cup of fresh cilantro, chopped
    7. 1/4 cup of roasted peanuts, chopped (optional)
    8. 3 tablespoons of rice vinegar
    9. 1 tablespoon of soy sauce
    10. 1 tablespoon of sesame oil

11. 1 teaspoon of honey (optional)

- **Instructions:**
  1. In a large bowl, combine the green cabbage, purple cabbage, carrot, bell pepper, green onions, and cilantro.
  2. In a small bowl, whisk together the rice vinegar, soy sauce, sesame oil, and honey.
  3. Pour the dressing over the salad and toss to combine.
  4. Sprinkle with roasted peanuts if desired and serve immediately.

2.1.3 Mexican Black Bean Salad

- **Prep Time:** 10 minutes
- **Cook Time:** 0 minutes
- **Servings:** 2
- **Ingredients:**
  1. 1 can of black beans, drained and rinsed
  2. 1 cup of corn kernels (fresh, canned, or frozen)
  3. 1 red bell pepper, diced
  4. 1/2 red onion, diced

5. 1 avocado, diced
6. 1/4 cup of fresh cilantro, chopped
7. Juice of 2 limes
8. 2 tablespoons of olive oil
9. 1 teaspoon of cumin
10. Salt and pepper to taste

- **Instructions:**
    1. In a large bowl, combine the black beans, corn, bell pepper, red onion, avocado, and cilantro.
    2. In a small bowl, whisk together the lime juice, olive oil, cumin, salt, and pepper.
    3. Pour the dressing over the salad and toss to combine.
    4. Serve immediately or refrigerate until ready to eat.

2.2 Hearty Soups and Stews

Soups and stews are perfect for a comforting, filling lunch. These no-point recipes are packed with flavor and nutrients to keep you satisfied throughout the day:

2.2.1 Classic Minestrone Soup

- **Prep Time:** 15 minutes
- **Cook Time:** 30 minutes
- **Servings:** 4
- **Ingredients:**
    1. 1 tablespoon of olive oil
    2. 1 onion, diced
    3. 2 cloves garlic, minced
    4. 2 carrots, diced
    5. 2 celery stalks, diced
    6. 1 zucchini, diced
    7. 1 can of diced tomatoes
    8. 1 can of kidney beans, drained and rinsed
    9. 4 cups of vegetable broth
    10. 1 teaspoon of dried oregano
    11. 1 teaspoon of dried basil
    12. 1/2 teaspoon of dried thyme
    13. Salt and pepper to taste
    14. 2 cups of fresh spinach
    15. 1/4 cup of fresh parsley, chopped

- **Instructions:**
    1. Heat the olive oil in a large pot over medium heat. Add the onion and garlic, cooking until softened (about 5 minutes).
    2. Add the carrots, celery, and zucchini, cooking for another 5 minutes.
    3. Stir in the diced tomatoes, kidney beans, vegetable broth, oregano, basil, thyme, salt, and pepper.
    4. Bring to a boil, then reduce heat and simmer for 20 minutes.
    5. Stir in the fresh spinach and cook until wilted (about 2 minutes).
    6. Garnish with fresh parsley and serve hot.

2.2.2 Lentil and Vegetable Stew

- **Prep Time:** 15 minutes
- **Cook Time:** 45 minutes
- **Servings:** 4
- **Ingredients:**
    1. 1 tablespoon of olive oil
    2. 1 onion, diced
    3. 2 cloves garlic, minced
    4. 2 carrots, diced
    5. 2 celery stalks, diced
    6. 1 sweet potato, diced
    7. 1 cup of dried green or brown lentils
    8. 4 cups of vegetable broth
    9. 1 can of diced tomatoes
    10. 1 teaspoon of ground cumin
    11. 1 teaspoon of ground coriander
    12. 1/2 teaspoon of smoked paprika
    13. Salt and pepper to taste
    14. 2 cups of kale, chopped
- **Instructions:**
    1. Heat the olive oil in a large pot over medium heat. Add the

onion and garlic, cooking until softened (about 5 minutes).

2. Add the carrots, celery, and sweet potato, cooking for another 5 minutes.

3. Stir in the lentils, vegetable broth, diced tomatoes, cumin, coriander, smoked paprika, salt, and pepper.

4. Bring to a boil, then reduce heat and simmer for 30 minutes, until the lentils and vegetables are tender.

5. Stir in the kale and cook until wilted (about 5 minutes).

6. Serve hot.

2.2.3 Chicken and Vegetable Soup

- **Prep Time:** 10 minutes
- **Cook Time:** 25 minutes
- **Servings:** 4
- **Ingredients:**
    1. 1 tablespoon of olive oil
    2. 1 onion, diced
    3. 2 cloves garlic, minced

4. 2 carrots, diced
5. 2 celery stalks, diced
6. 2 cups of shredded cooked chicken breast
7. 4 cups of chicken broth
8. 1 can of diced tomatoes
9. 1 teaspoon of dried thyme
10. 1 teaspoon of dried basil
11. Salt and pepper to taste
12. 2 cups of baby spinach

- **Instructions:**
  1. Heat the olive oil in a large pot over medium heat. Add the onion and garlic, cooking until softened (about 5 minutes).
  2. Add the carrots and celery, cooking for another 5 minutes.
  3. Stir in the shredded chicken, chicken broth, diced tomatoes, thyme, basil, salt, and pepper.
  4. Bring to a boil, then reduce heat and simmer for 15 minutes.
  5. Stir in the baby spinach and cook until wilted (about 2 minutes).

6. Serve hot.

2.3 Light and Delicious Wraps and Sandwiches

Wraps and sandwiches are perfect for a quick and easy lunch. Here are some no-point options that are both light and delicious:

2.3.1 Turkey and Avocado Wrap

- **Prep Time:** 5 minutes
- **Cook Time:** 0 minutes
- **Servings:** 1
- **Ingredients:**
    1. 1 whole-grain wrap
    2. 3 slices of lean turkey breast
    3. 1/2 avocado, sliced
    4. 1/4 cup of shredded lettuce
    5. 1/4 cup of diced tomatoes
    6. 1 tablespoon of Greek yogurt
    7. Salt and pepper to taste
- **Instructions:**
    1. Lay the whole-grain wrap flat on a plate.

2. Spread the Greek yogurt over the wrap.
3. Layer the turkey, avocado, lettuce, and tomatoes on top.
4. Season with salt and pepper.
5. Roll up the wrap tightly and slice in half.

2.3.2 Hummus and Veggie Sandwich

- **Prep Time:** 10 minutes
- **Cook Time:** 0 minutes
- **Servings:** 1
- **Ingredients:**
    1. 2 slices of whole-grain bread
    2. 1/4 cup of hummus
    3. 1/2 cucumber, sliced
    4. 1/4 red bell pepper, sliced
    5. 1/4 cup of shredded carrots
    6. 1/4 cup of alfalfa sprouts
    7. Salt and pepper to taste
- **Instructions:**
    1. Spread the hummus on both slices of whole-grain bread.

2. Layer the cucumber, bell pepper, carrots, and alfalfa sprouts on one slice.
3. Season with salt and pepper.
4. Top with the other slice of bread and cut in half.

2.3.3 Tuna Salad Lettuce Wraps

- **Prep Time:** 10 minutes
- **Cook Time:** 0 minutes
- **Servings:** 1
- **Ingredients:**
    1. 1 can of tuna, drained
    2. 1 tablespoon of Greek yogurt
    3. 1 teaspoon of Dijon mustard
    4. 1 celery stalk, diced
    5. 1/4 red onion, diced
    6. Salt and pepper to taste
    7. 4 large lettuce leaves
- **Instructions:**
    1. In a bowl, combine the tuna, Greek yogurt, Dijon mustard, celery, red onion, salt, and pepper.

2. Spoon the tuna mixture onto the lettuce leaves.

3. Roll up the lettuce leaves and serve.

2.4 Meal Prep Tips for Easy Lunchtime Solutions

Meal prepping is a great way to ensure you have healthy, no-point lunches ready to go. Here are some tips to make meal prep easier and more efficient:

2.4.1 Plan Your Menu

- Take some time at the beginning of each week to plan your lunches. Choose recipes that you can prepare in advance and that will keep well in the fridge.

2.4.2 Batch Cooking

- Cook large batches of soups, stews, and grains that you can portion out for several meals. This saves time and ensures you always have a healthy option on hand.

2.4.3 Use Quality Storage Containers

- Invest in a set of good quality, airtight storage containers. These will keep your meals fresh and make it easy to grab and go.

2.4.4 Prep Ingredients in Advance

- Chop vegetables, cook proteins, and prepare dressings ahead of time. Store them separately and assemble your lunches each day to keep everything fresh.

2.4.5 Label and Date Your Meals

- Label your containers with the name of the dish and the date it was prepared. This helps you keep track of what's in your fridge and ensures you eat everything before it spoils.

With these recipes and tips, you'll have no trouble enjoying satisfying and nutritious no-point lunches every day. Enjoy these delicious options and feel great knowing you're nourishing your body with healthy, flavorful meals!

Chapter 3: Delicious Dinners

Dinner is a time to relax and enjoy a satisfying meal after a busy day. With these no-point recipes, you can prepare delicious dinners that are both healthy and easy to make. Whether you need a quick one-pot meal, a flavorful main course, vegetarian and vegan options, or something the whole family will love, this chapter has you covered.

3.1 One-Pot Meals for Busy Weeknights

One-pot meals are perfect for busy weeknights when you want a quick and easy dinner with minimal cleanup. Here are some no-point one-pot meals to add to your dinner rotation:

3.1.1 Chicken and Vegetable Stir-Fry

- **Prep Time:** 10 minutes
- **Cook Time:** 15 minutes
- **Servings:** 4
- **Ingredients:**
    1. 1 tablespoon of olive oil
    2. 2 boneless, skinless chicken breasts, cut into strips
    3. 1 red bell pepper, sliced
    4. 1 yellow bell pepper, sliced
    5. 1 cup of snap peas
    6. 1 cup of broccoli florets
    7. 2 cloves garlic, minced
    8. 1 tablespoon of soy sauce
    9. 1 tablespoon of hoisin sauce
    10. 1 teaspoon of sesame oil
    11. 1 teaspoon of grated ginger
- **Instructions:**
    1. Heat the olive oil in a large skillet or wok over medium-high heat.
    2. Add the chicken strips and cook until browned (about 5 minutes).

3. Add the bell peppers, snap peas, broccoli, and garlic, cooking for another 5 minutes.
4. Stir in the soy sauce, hoisin sauce, sesame oil, and grated ginger.
5. Cook for an additional 5 minutes, until the vegetables are tender.
6. Serve hot.

3.1.2 Beef and Quinoa Stuffed Peppers

- **Prep Time:** 15 minutes
- **Cook Time:** 30 minutes
- **Servings:** 4
- **Ingredients:**
  1. 4 large bell peppers, tops cut off and seeds removed
  2. 1 pound of lean ground beef
  3. 1 cup of cooked quinoa
  4. 1 can of diced tomatoes
  5. 1 cup of black beans, drained and rinsed
  6. 1 teaspoon of cumin
  7. 1 teaspoon of chili powder

8. Salt and pepper to taste

9. 1/2 cup of shredded cheese (optional)

- **Instructions:**

    1. Preheat the oven to 375°F (190°C).

    2. In a large skillet, cook the ground beef over medium heat until browned.

    3. Stir in the cooked quinoa, diced tomatoes, black beans, cumin, chili powder, salt, and pepper.

    4. Stuff the bell peppers with the beef and quinoa mixture.

    5. Place the stuffed peppers in a baking dish and bake for 30 minutes.

    6. Top with shredded cheese, if desired, and serve hot.

3.1.3 Shrimp and Vegetable Paella

- **Prep Time:** 15 minutes
- **Cook Time:** 30 minutes
- **Servings:** 4
- **Ingredients:**

1. 1 tablespoon of olive oil
2. 1 onion, diced
3. 2 cloves garlic, minced
4. 1 red bell pepper, diced
5. 1 cup of green beans, chopped
6. 1 cup of cherry tomatoes, halved
7. 1 cup of Arborio rice
8. 4 cups of chicken or vegetable broth
9. 1 teaspoon of smoked paprika
10. 1/2 teaspoon of saffron threads (optional)
11. Salt and pepper to taste
12. 1 pound of shrimp, peeled and deveined
13. 1/4 cup of fresh parsley, chopped

- **Instructions:**
  1. Heat the olive oil in a large skillet over medium heat.
  2. Add the onion and garlic, cooking until softened (about 5 minutes).

3. Stir in the bell pepper, green beans, and cherry tomatoes, cooking for another 5 minutes.

4. Add the Arborio rice and cook for 2 minutes, stirring constantly.

5. Pour in the chicken or vegetable broth, smoked paprika, saffron, salt, and pepper.

6. Bring to a boil, then reduce heat and simmer for 20 minutes, stirring occasionally.

7. Add the shrimp and cook until they are pink and cooked through (about 5 minutes).

8. Garnish with fresh parsley and serve hot.

3.2 Flavorful No-Point Main Courses

Main courses can be both flavorful and healthy. Here are some no-point main courses that are sure to please your palate:

3.2.1 Lemon Herb Grilled Chicken

- **Prep Time:** 10 minutes (plus 30 minutes marinating time)
- **Cook Time:** 15 minutes
- **Servings:** 4
- **Ingredients:**
  1. 4 boneless, skinless chicken breasts
  2. Juice of 2 lemons
  3. 2 tablespoons of olive oil
  4. 2 cloves garlic, minced
  5. 1 tablespoon of fresh thyme, chopped
  6. 1 tablespoon of fresh rosemary, chopped
  7. Salt and pepper to taste

- **Instructions:**
    1. In a bowl, combine the lemon juice, olive oil, garlic, thyme, rosemary, salt, and pepper.
    2. Place the chicken breasts in a resealable plastic bag and pour the marinade over them.
    3. Marinate in the refrigerator for at least 30 minutes.
    4. Preheat the grill to medium-high heat.
    5. Grill the chicken breasts for 6-8 minutes on each side, until fully cooked.
    6. Serve hot with a side of vegetables or salad.

3.2.2 Baked Salmon with Dill and Lemon

- **Prep Time:** 10 minutes
- **Cook Time:** 20 minutes
- **Servings:** 4
- **Ingredients:**
    1. 4 salmon fillets
    2. 2 tablespoons of olive oil
    3. Juice of 1 lemon

4. 2 tablespoons of fresh dill, chopped
5. Salt and pepper to taste

- **Instructions:**
  1. Preheat the oven to 375°F (190°C).
  2. Place the salmon fillets on a baking sheet lined with parchment paper.
  3. Drizzle with olive oil and lemon juice.
  4. Sprinkle with fresh dill, salt, and pepper.
  5. Bake for 20 minutes, until the salmon is cooked through and flakes easily with a fork.
  6. Serve hot with a side of roasted vegetables.

3.2.3 Spicy Tofu Stir-Fry

- **Prep Time:** 10 minutes
- **Cook Time:** 15 minutes
- **Servings:** 4
- **Ingredients:**
    1. 1 tablespoon of sesame oil
    2. 1 block of firm tofu, pressed and cubed
    3. 1 red bell pepper, sliced
    4. 1 green bell pepper, sliced
    5. 1 cup of snap peas
    6. 2 cloves garlic, minced
    7. 1 tablespoon of soy sauce
    8. 1 tablespoon of hoisin sauce
    9. 1 teaspoon of sriracha sauce (optional)
    10. 1 teaspoon of grated ginger
- **Instructions:**
    1. Heat the sesame oil in a large skillet or wok over medium-high heat.
    2. Add the cubed tofu and cook until golden brown on all sides (about 5 minutes).

3. Remove the tofu from the skillet and set aside.
4. Add the bell peppers, snap peas, and garlic to the skillet, cooking for 5 minutes.
5. Stir in the soy sauce, hoisin sauce, sriracha sauce, and grated ginger.
6. Return the tofu to the skillet and cook for an additional 5 minutes.
7. Serve hot with a side of steamed rice.

3.3 Vegetarian and Vegan Dinner Options

Vegetarian and vegan dinners can be just as satisfying and flavorful as their meat-based counterparts. Here are some no-point options to try:

3.3.1 Quinoa and Black Bean Stuffed Sweet Potatoes

- **Prep Time:** 10 minutes
- **Cook Time:** 45 minutes
- **Servings:** 4
- **Ingredients:**
    1. 4 large sweet potatoes
    2. 1 cup of cooked quinoa
    3. 1 can of black beans, drained and rinsed
    4. 1 cup of corn kernels (fresh, canned, or frozen)
    5. 1/4 cup of fresh cilantro, chopped
    6. Juice of 2 limes
    7. 1 teaspoon of cumin
    8. Salt and pepper to taste
    9. 1/2 cup of avocado, diced
- **Instructions:**
    1. Preheat the oven to 400°F (200°C).
    2. Pierce the sweet potatoes with a fork and bake for 45 minutes, until tender.

3. In a bowl, combine the cooked quinoa, black beans, corn, cilantro, lime juice, cumin, salt, and pepper.
4. Once the sweet potatoes are cooked, cut them in half and scoop out a portion of the flesh.
5. Stuff the sweet potatoes with the quinoa and black bean mixture.
6. Top with diced avocado and serve hot.

3.3.2 Lentil and Vegetable Curry

- **Prep Time:** 10 minutes
- **Cook Time:** 30 minutes
- **Servings:** 4
- **Ingredients:**
  1. 1 tablespoon of coconut oil
  2. 1 onion, diced
  3. 2 cloves garlic, minced
  4. 1 tablespoon of grated ginger
  5. 2 carrots, diced
  6. 1 red bell pepper, diced
  7. 1 cup of dried lentils

8. 1 can of coconut milk

9. 2 cups of vegetable broth

10. 1 tablespoon of curry powder

11. 1 teaspoon of turmeric

12. Salt and pepper to taste

13. 2 cups of fresh spinach

- **Instructions:**

    1. Heat the coconut oil in a large pot over medium heat.

    2. Add the onion, garlic, and ginger, cooking until softened (about 5 minutes).

    3. Stir in the carrots and bell pepper, cooking for another 5 minutes.

    4. Add the dried lentils, coconut milk, vegetable broth, curry powder, turmeric, salt, and pepper.

    5. Bring to a boil, then reduce heat and simmer for 20 minutes, until the lentils are tender.

    6. Stir in the fresh spinach and cook until wilted (about 2 minutes).

7. Serve hot with a side of rice or naan bread.

3.3.3 Spaghetti Squash with Marinara Sauce

- **Prep Time:** 10 minutes
- **Cook Time:** 40 minutes
- **Servings:** 4
- **Ingredients:**
  1. 1 large spaghetti squash
  2. 1 tablespoon of olive oil
  3. 1 onion, diced
  4. 2 cloves garlic, minced
  5. 1 can of crushed tomatoes
  6. 1 teaspoon of dried oregano
  7. 1 teaspoon of dried basil
  8. Salt and pepper to taste
  9. 1/4 cup of fresh parsley, chopped
- **Instructions:**
  1. Preheat the oven to 375°F (190°C).
  2. Cut the spaghetti squash in half lengthwise and remove the seeds.

3. Place the squash halves cut-side down on a baking sheet and bake for 40 minutes, until tender.
4. While the squash is baking, heat the olive oil in a saucepan over medium heat.
5. Add the onion and garlic, cooking until softened (about 5 minutes).
6. Stir in the crushed tomatoes, oregano, basil, salt, and pepper.
7. Simmer the sauce for 20 minutes.
8. Once the squash is cooked, use a fork to scrape the flesh into strands.
9. Serve the spaghetti squash topped with marinara sauce and fresh parsley.

3.4 Family-Friendly Dinner Ideas

These no-point dinner recipes are perfect for the whole family. They are tasty, healthy, and easy to prepare:

3.4.1 Turkey Meatballs with Zucchini Noodles

- **Prep Time:** 15 minutes
- **Cook Time:** 20 minutes
- **Servings:** 4
- **Ingredients:**
    1. 1 pound of ground turkey
    2. 1/4 cup of breadcrumbs
    3. 1/4 cup of grated Parmesan cheese
    4. 1 egg
    5. 2 cloves garlic, minced
    6. 1 tablespoon of fresh parsley, chopped
    7. Salt and pepper to taste
    8. 4 large zucchinis, spiralized
    9. 1 jar of marinara sauce

- **Instructions:**
  1. Preheat the oven to 375°F (190°C).
  2. In a bowl, combine the ground turkey, breadcrumbs, Parmesan cheese, egg, garlic, parsley, salt, and pepper.
  3. Form the mixture into meatballs and place them on a baking sheet.
  4. Bake for 20 minutes, until fully cooked.
  5. While the meatballs are baking, heat the marinara sauce in a saucepan over medium heat.
  6. Add the spiralized zucchini noodles to the sauce and cook for 5 minutes, until tender.
  7. Serve the meatballs on top of the zucchini noodles.

3.4.2 Baked Chicken Parmesan

- **Prep Time:** 10 minutes
- **Cook Time:** 25 minutes
- **Servings:** 4
- **Ingredients:**
    1. 4 boneless, skinless chicken breasts
    2. 1 cup of breadcrumbs
    3. 1/2 cup of grated Parmesan cheese
    4. 1 egg, beaten
    5. 1 jar of marinara sauce
    6. 1/2 cup of shredded mozzarella cheese
    7. Salt and pepper to taste
- **Instructions:**
    1. Preheat the oven to 375°F (190°C).
    2. In a bowl, combine the breadcrumbs, Parmesan cheese, salt, and pepper.
    3. Dip the chicken breasts in the beaten egg, then coat with the breadcrumb mixture.

4. Place the chicken breasts on a baking sheet and bake for 20 minutes.
5. Remove the chicken from the oven and top each breast with marinara sauce and mozzarella cheese.
6. Return to the oven and bake for an additional 5 minutes, until the cheese is melted.
7. Serve hot with a side of vegetables or salad.

3.4.3 Veggie-Packed Mac and Cheese

- **Prep Time:** 10 minutes
- **Cook Time:** 20 minutes
- **Servings:** 4
- **Ingredients:**
  1. 8 ounces of whole-grain macaroni
  2. 1 tablespoon of olive oil
  3. 1 onion, diced
  4. 2 cloves garlic, minced
  5. 1 cup of broccoli florets
  6. 1 cup of diced carrots

7. 1 cup of peas
8. 1 cup of shredded cheddar cheese
9. 1 cup of non-fat Greek yogurt
10. Salt and pepper to taste

- **Instructions:**
  1. Cook the macaroni according to package instructions.
  2. While the pasta is cooking, heat the olive oil in a large skillet over medium heat.
  3. Add the onion and garlic, cooking until softened (about 5 minutes).
  4. Stir in the broccoli, carrots, and peas, cooking for another 5 minutes.
  5. Drain the macaroni and return it to the pot.
  6. Stir in the cooked vegetables, cheddar cheese, Greek yogurt, salt, and pepper.
  7. Cook over low heat until the cheese is melted and everything is well combined.

8. Serve hot.

With these no-point dinner recipes, you can enjoy delicious, healthy meals every night of the week. Whether you're cooking for yourself, your family, or entertaining guests, these dishes are sure to satisfy. Enjoy these flavorful options and feel great knowing you're nourishing your body with wholesome, nutritious foods!

Chapter 4: Snacks and Appetizers

Snacks and appetizers are an essential part of any diet, providing quick energy boosts and satisfying hunger between meals. With these no-point recipes, you can enjoy tasty and healthy snacks and appetizers without any guilt. This chapter offers a variety of options, from quick snacks to delicious dips and satisfying appetizers perfect for entertaining.

4.1 Quick No-Point Snacks for On-the-Go

When you're on the go and need a quick bite, these no-point snacks are perfect for keeping you fueled and satisfied:

4.1.1 Fresh Veggie Sticks

- **Prep Time:** 10 minutes
- **Cook Time:** 0 minutes
- **Servings:** 4
- **Ingredients:**
    1. 2 carrots, peeled and cut into sticks
    2. 2 celery stalks, cut into sticks
    3. 1 cucumber, sliced into sticks
    4. 1 red bell pepper, sliced into sticks
    5. 1 cup of cherry tomatoes
- **Instructions:**
    1. Prepare all the vegetables by washing, peeling, and cutting them into sticks.
    2. Arrange the veggie sticks and cherry tomatoes in a container for easy snacking.
    3. Enjoy with your favorite no-point dip or on their own.

4.1.2 Hard-Boiled Eggs

- **Prep Time:** 5 minutes
- **Cook Time:** 10 minutes
- **Servings:** 6
- **Ingredients:**
    1. 6 eggs
- **Instructions:**
    1. Place the eggs in a pot and cover with cold water.
    2. Bring to a boil, then reduce the heat and simmer for 10 minutes.
    3. Remove from the heat and let cool.
    4. Peel the eggs and store in the refrigerator for a quick protein-packed snack.

4.1.3 Apple Slices with Almond Butter

- **Prep Time:** 5 minutes
- **Cook Time:** 0 minutes
- **Servings:** 2
- **Ingredients:**
    1. 2 apples, cored and sliced
    2. 2 tablespoons of almond butter
- **Instructions:**
    1. Slice the apples and arrange them on a plate.
    2. Serve with almond butter for dipping.
    3. Enjoy as a quick and nutritious snack.

4.2 Healthy Dips and Spreads

Dips and spreads are great for pairing with fresh veggies, whole-grain crackers, or even spreading on sandwiches. Here are some healthy, no-point options:

4.2.1 Classic Hummus

- **Prep Time:** 10 minutes
- **Cook Time:** 0 minutes
- **Servings:** 4
- **Ingredients:**
  1. 1 can of chickpeas, drained and rinsed
  2. 1/4 cup of tahini
  3. Juice of 1 lemon
  4. 2 cloves garlic
  5. 2 tablespoons of olive oil
  6. 1/2 teaspoon of cumin
  7. Salt and pepper to taste
  8. Water, as needed
- **Instructions:**
  1. In a food processor, combine the chickpeas, tahini, lemon juice, garlic, olive oil, cumin, salt, and pepper.
  2. Blend until smooth, adding water as needed to reach the desired consistency.
  3. Serve with fresh veggies or whole-grain crackers.

4.2.2 Guacamole

- **Prep Time:** 10 minutes
- **Cook Time:** 0 minutes
- **Servings:** 4
- **Ingredients:**
    1. 3 ripe avocados
    2. Juice of 2 limes
    3. 1 small red onion, finely chopped
    4. 1 tomato, diced
    5. 1/4 cup of fresh cilantro, chopped
    6. 1 jalapeno, minced (optional)
    7. Salt and pepper to taste
- **Instructions:**
    1. In a bowl, mash the avocados with lime juice until smooth.
    2. Stir in the red onion, tomato, cilantro, jalapeno (if using), salt, and pepper.
    3. Serve with veggie sticks or whole-grain chips.

4.2.3 Greek Yogurt Tzatziki

- **Prep Time:** 10 minutes
- **Cook Time:** 0 minutes
- **Servings:** 4
- **Ingredients:**
  1. 1 cup of non-fat Greek yogurt
  2. 1/2 cucumber, grated and squeezed of excess water
  3. 2 cloves garlic, minced
  4. Juice of 1 lemon
  5. 1 tablespoon of olive oil
  6. 1 tablespoon of fresh dill, chopped
  7. Salt and pepper to taste
- **Instructions:**
  1. In a bowl, combine the Greek yogurt, grated cucumber, garlic, lemon juice, olive oil, dill, salt, and pepper.
  2. Mix well and refrigerate for at least 30 minutes before serving.
  3. Serve with veggie sticks or pita bread.

4.3 Guilt-Free Appetizers for Entertaining

Hosting a party or gathering? These guilt-free appetizers are perfect for entertaining without compromising on taste:

4.3.1 Caprese Skewers

- **Prep Time:** 10 minutes
- **Cook Time:** 0 minutes
- **Servings:** 4
- **Ingredients:**
    1. 1 pint of cherry tomatoes
    2. 1 small container of mozzarella balls
    3. Fresh basil leaves
    4. Balsamic glaze (optional)
- **Instructions:**
    1. Thread a cherry tomato, a mozzarella ball, and a basil leaf onto small skewers or toothpicks.
    2. Arrange on a platter and drizzle with balsamic glaze if desired.
    3. Serve immediately.

4.3.2 Stuffed Mini Bell Peppers

- **Prep Time:** 15 minutes
- **Cook Time:** 0 minutes
- **Servings:** 4
- **Ingredients:**
    1. 12 mini bell peppers, halved and seeded
    2. 1 cup of non-fat Greek yogurt
    3. 1/2 cup of crumbled feta cheese
    4. 2 tablespoons of fresh dill, chopped
    5. 1 tablespoon of lemon juice
    6. Salt and pepper to taste
- **Instructions:**
    1. In a bowl, mix the Greek yogurt, feta cheese, dill, lemon juice, salt, and pepper.
    2. Stuff each bell pepper half with the mixture.
    3. Arrange on a platter and serve immediately.

4.3.3 Cucumber Bites with Smoked Salmon

- **Prep Time:** 10 minutes
- **Cook Time:** 0 minutes
- **Servings:** 4
- **Ingredients:**
    1. 1 large cucumber, sliced into rounds
    2. 4 ounces of smoked salmon, cut into small pieces
    3. 1/4 cup of non-fat Greek yogurt
    4. 1 tablespoon of capers
    5. Fresh dill for garnish
- **Instructions:**
    1. Arrange the cucumber slices on a serving platter.
    2. Top each slice with a small piece of smoked salmon.
    3. Add a dollop of Greek yogurt on top and garnish with capers and fresh dill.
    4. Serve immediately.

4.4 Crunchy and Satisfying Snack Recipes

When you're craving something crunchy and satisfying, these no-point snacks will hit the spot:

4.4.1 Roasted Chickpeas

- **Prep Time:** 10 minutes
- **Cook Time:** 30 minutes
- **Servings:** 4
- **Ingredients:**
    1. 1 can of chickpeas, drained and rinsed
    2. 1 tablespoon of olive oil
    3. 1 teaspoon of smoked paprika
    4. 1/2 teaspoon of garlic powder
    5. Salt and pepper to taste
- **Instructions:**
    1. Preheat the oven to 400°F (200°C).
    2. Pat the chickpeas dry with a paper towel.
    3. In a bowl, toss the chickpeas with olive oil, smoked paprika, garlic powder, salt, and pepper.

4. Spread the chickpeas on a baking sheet in a single layer.
5. Roast for 30 minutes, shaking the pan halfway through, until crispy.
6. Allow to cool slightly before serving.

4.4.2 Baked Zucchini Chips

- **Prep Time:** 10 minutes
- **Cook Time:** 20 minutes
- **Servings:** 4
- **Ingredients:**
  1. 2 zucchinis, thinly sliced
  2. 1 tablespoon of olive oil
  3. 1 teaspoon of Italian seasoning
  4. Salt and pepper to taste
- **Instructions:**
  1. Preheat the oven to 375°F (190°C).
  2. In a bowl, toss the zucchini slices with olive oil, Italian seasoning, salt, and pepper.
  3. Arrange the zucchini slices on a baking sheet in a single layer.

4. Bake for 20 minutes, until golden brown and crispy.
5. Allow to cool slightly before serving.

4.4.3 Spiced Almonds

- **Prep Time:** 5 minutes
- **Cook Time:** 10 minutes
- **Servings:** 4
- **Ingredients:**
    1. 1 cup of raw almonds
    2. 1 tablespoon of olive oil
    3. 1 teaspoon of chili powder
    4. 1/2 teaspoon of cumin
    5. 1/2 teaspoon of smoked paprika
    6. Salt to taste
- **Instructions:**
    1. Preheat the oven to 350°F (175°C).
    2. In a bowl, toss the almonds with olive oil, chili powder, cumin, smoked paprika, and salt.
    3. Spread the almonds on a baking sheet in a single layer.

4. Bake for 10 minutes, stirring halfway through, until toasted and fragrant.
5. Allow to cool slightly before serving.

With these no-point snacks and appetizers, you can enjoy tasty, healthy options throughout the day and for any occasion. Whether you're looking for something quick and easy, or a dish to impress your guests, these recipes have you covered. Enjoy these guilt-free options and feel great knowing you're making nutritious choices!

Chapter 5: Smoothies

Smoothies are an excellent way to pack a lot of nutrients into one delicious drink. They can be a quick breakfast, a post-workout recovery drink, or a refreshing snack. This chapter focuses on no-point smoothies that are both refreshing and nutritious, ensuring you get the best of both worlds.

5.1 Refreshing No-Point Smoothies

These no-point smoothies are designed to be both delicious and healthy, perfect for any time of the day.

5.1.1 Green Detox Smoothie

- **Prep Time:** 5 minutes
- **Cook Time:** 0 minutes
- **Servings:** 1
- **Ingredients:**
    1. 1 cup of spinach
    2. 1/2 cucumber, chopped
    3. 1 green apple, cored and chopped

4. 1/2 lemon, juiced
5. 1 cup of water or coconut water
6. Ice cubes (optional)

- **Instructions:**
    1. Place all ingredients in a blender.
    2. Blend until smooth.
    3. Pour into a glass and enjoy immediately.

5.1.2 Berry Blast Smoothie

- **Prep Time:** 5 minutes
- **Cook Time:** 0 minutes
- **Servings:** 1
- **Ingredients:**
    1. 1 cup of mixed berries (strawberries, blueberries, raspberries)
    2. 1/2 banana
    3. 1 cup of unsweetened almond milk
    4. 1 tablespoon of chia seeds
- **Instructions:**
    1. Place all ingredients in a blender.

2. Blend until smooth.
3. Pour into a glass and enjoy immediately.

5.1.3 Tropical Delight Smoothie

- **Prep Time:** 5 minutes
- **Cook Time:** 0 minutes
- **Servings:** 1
- **Ingredients:**
    1. 1 cup of pineapple chunks
    2. 1/2 mango, peeled and chopped
    3. 1/2 banana
    4. 1 cup of coconut water
    5. Ice cubes (optional)
- **Instructions:**
    1. Place all ingredients in a blender.
    2. Blend until smooth.
    3. Pour into a glass and enjoy immediately.

5.1.4 Peanut Butter Banana Smoothie

- **Prep Time:** 5 minutes
- **Cook Time:** 0 minutes
- **Servings:** 1
- **Ingredients:**
    1. 1 banana
    2. 1 tablespoon of natural peanut butter
    3. 1 cup of unsweetened almond milk
    4. 1 tablespoon of flax seeds
- **Instructions:**
    1. Place all ingredients in a blender.
    2. Blend until smooth.
    3. Pour into a glass and enjoy immediately.

5.1.5 Orange Creamsicle Smoothie

- **Prep Time:** 5 minutes
- **Cook Time:** 0 minutes
- **Servings:** 1
- **Ingredients:**
    1. 1 orange, peeled and segmented
    2. 1/2 cup of unsweetened almond milk
    3. 1/2 cup of non-fat Greek yogurt
    4. 1 teaspoon of vanilla extract
    5. Ice cubes (optional)
- **Instructions:**
    1. Place all ingredients in a blender.
    2. Blend until smooth.
    3. Pour into a glass and enjoy immediately.

5.1.6 Green Tea Smoothie

- **Prep Time:** 5 minutes
- **Cook Time:** 0 minutes
- **Servings:** 1
- **Ingredients:**
  1. 1 cup of brewed green tea, cooled
  2. 1/2 cup of spinach
  3. 1/2 avocado
  4. 1/2 apple, cored and chopped
  5. 1 tablespoon of lemon juice
  6. Ice cubes (optional)
- **Instructions:**
  1. Place all ingredients in a blender.
  2. Blend until smooth.
  3. Pour into a glass and enjoy immediately.

5.1.7 Chocolate Banana Smoothie

- **Prep Time:** 5 minutes
- **Cook Time:** 0 minutes
- **Servings:** 1
- **Ingredients:**

1. 1 banana
2. 1 tablespoon of unsweetened cocoa powder
3. 1 cup of unsweetened almond milk
4. 1 tablespoon of chia seeds

- **Instructions:**
    1. Place all ingredients in a blender.
    2. Blend until smooth.
    3. Pour into a glass and enjoy immediately.

5.1.8 Strawberry Kiwi Smoothie

- **Prep Time:** 5 minutes
- **Cook Time:** 0 minutes
- **Servings:** 1
- **Ingredients:**
    1. 1 cup of strawberries, hulled
    2. 2 kiwis, peeled and chopped
    3. 1 cup of unsweetened almond milk
    4. 1 tablespoon of flax seeds

- **Instructions:**
    1. Place all ingredients in a blender.
    2. Blend until smooth.
    3. Pour into a glass and enjoy immediately.

5.1.9 Blueberry Spinach Smoothie

- **Prep Time:** 5 minutes
- **Cook Time:** 0 minutes
- **Servings:** 1
- **Ingredients:**
    1. 1 cup of blueberries
    2. 1 cup of spinach
    3. 1/2 banana
    4. 1 cup of unsweetened almond milk
    5. 1 tablespoon of chia seeds
- **Instructions:**
    1. Place all ingredients in a blender.
    2. Blend until smooth.
    3. Pour into a glass and enjoy immediately.

5.1.10 Pineapple Mint Smoothie

- **Prep Time:** 5 minutes
- **Cook Time:** 0 minutes
- **Servings:** 1
- **Ingredients:**
    1. 1 cup of pineapple chunks
    2. 1/2 cucumber, chopped
    3. 1/4 cup of fresh mint leaves
    4. 1 cup of coconut water
    5. Ice cubes (optional)
- **Instructions:**
    1. Place all ingredients in a blender.
    2. Blend until smooth.
    3. Pour into a glass and enjoy immediately.

These no-point smoothies are not only refreshing and delicious but also packed with nutrients to keep you energized and satisfied. Enjoy these recipes as a quick breakfast, a post-workout drink, or a healthy snack any time of the day!

Chapter 6: Desserts

Desserts can be a delightful part of a healthy eating plan when made with nutritious ingredients. This chapter features no-point desserts that are both delicious and guilt-free. From fruit-based treats to no-bake sweets and indulgent yet healthy options, these recipes will satisfy your sweet tooth without compromising your diet.

6.1 Fruit-Based Desserts

Fruit-based desserts are naturally sweet and packed with nutrients. Here are some no-point options to enjoy:

6.1.1 Baked Apples with Cinnamon

- **Prep Time:** 10 minutes
- **Cook Time:** 30 minutes
- **Servings:** 4
- **Ingredients:**
    1. 4 apples, cored
    2. 1 teaspoon of ground cinnamon
    3. 1/4 cup of raisins

4. 1/4 cup of chopped nuts (optional)

- **Instructions:**
  1. Preheat the oven to 375°F (190°C).
  2. Place the cored apples in a baking dish.
  3. Sprinkle the cinnamon inside the apples.
  4. Stuff the apples with raisins and nuts, if using.
  5. Bake for 30 minutes, until the apples are tender.
  6. Serve warm.

6.1.2 Grilled Pineapple with Lime

- **Prep Time:** 5 minutes
- **Cook Time:** 10 minutes
- **Servings:** 4
- **Ingredients:**
  1. 1 pineapple, peeled, cored, and cut into rings
  2. Juice of 2 limes
  3. 1 tablespoon of honey (optional)

- **Instructions:**
    1. Preheat the grill to medium-high heat.
    2. Brush the pineapple rings with lime juice and honey, if using.
    3. Grill the pineapple for 2-3 minutes on each side, until grill marks appear.
    4. Serve warm or chilled.

6.1.3 Berry Parfait

- **Prep Time:** 10 minutes
- **Cook Time:** 0 minutes
- **Servings:** 2
- **Ingredients:**
    1. 1 cup of mixed berries (strawberries, blueberries, raspberries)
    2. 1 cup of non-fat Greek yogurt
    3. 1 tablespoon of honey (optional)
    4. Fresh mint leaves for garnish

- **Instructions:**
    1. In a glass or bowl, layer the Greek yogurt and mixed berries.
    2. Drizzle with honey, if using.
    3. Garnish with fresh mint leaves.
    4. Serve immediately.

6.2 No-Bake Treats and Sweets

No-bake desserts are quick and easy to prepare, perfect for satisfying your sweet cravings without the need for an oven:

6.2.1 Chocolate Banana Bites

- **Prep Time:** 10 minutes
- **Cook Time:** 0 minutes (plus 1 hour freezing time)
- **Servings:** 4
- **Ingredients:**
    1. 2 bananas, sliced into rounds
    2. 1/2 cup of dark chocolate chips, melted
    3. 1/4 cup of chopped nuts (optional)

- **Instructions:**
    1. Dip each banana slice into the melted dark chocolate.
    2. Place the chocolate-covered banana slices on a baking sheet lined with parchment paper.
    3. Sprinkle with chopped nuts, if using.
    4. Freeze for at least 1 hour.
    5. Serve frozen.

6.2.2 Peanut Butter Energy Balls

- **Prep Time:** 10 minutes
- **Cook Time:** 0 minutes
- **Servings:** 12 balls
- **Ingredients:**
    1. 1 cup of oats
    2. 1/2 cup of natural peanut butter
    3. 1/4 cup of honey
    4. 1/4 cup of flax seeds
    5. 1/4 cup of dark chocolate chips (optional)
- **Instructions:**
    1. In a bowl, combine the oats, peanut butter, honey, flax seeds,

and dark chocolate chips, if using.
2. Mix well until combined.
3. Roll the mixture into small balls.
4. Refrigerate for at least 30 minutes before serving.

6.2.3 No-Bake Cheesecake Cups

- **Prep Time:** 15 minutes
- **Cook Time:** 0 minutes
- **Servings:** 4
- **Ingredients:**
    1. 1 cup of non-fat Greek yogurt
    2. 1/4 cup of low-fat cream cheese
    3. 1 tablespoon of honey
    4. 1/2 teaspoon of vanilla extract
    5. 1/2 cup of crushed graham crackers (optional)
    6. Fresh berries for topping
- **Instructions:**
    1. In a bowl, beat together the Greek yogurt, cream cheese, honey, and vanilla extract until smooth.

2. Divide the mixture into small cups or ramekins.
3. Top with crushed graham crackers, if using, and fresh berries.
4. Refrigerate for at least 1 hour before serving.

6.3 Indulgent yet Healthy Dessert Options

These indulgent yet healthy desserts offer the perfect balance of taste and nutrition, making them a great choice for any occasion:

6.3.1 Dark Chocolate Avocado Mousse

- **Prep Time:** 10 minutes
- **Cook Time:** 0 minutes
- **Servings:** 4
- **Ingredients:**
  1. 2 ripe avocados
  2. 1/4 cup of unsweetened cocoa powder
  3. 1/4 cup of honey
  4. 1/4 cup of almond milk

5. 1 teaspoon of vanilla extract
6. Fresh berries for topping

- **Instructions:**
  1. In a blender, combine the avocados, cocoa powder, honey, almond milk, and vanilla extract.
  2. Blend until smooth and creamy.
  3. Divide the mousse into small bowls or cups.
  4. Top with fresh berries.
  5. Refrigerate for at least 30 minutes before serving.

6.3.2 Chia Seed Pudding

- **Prep Time:** 10 minutes (plus overnight chilling)
- **Cook Time:** 0 minutes
- **Servings:** 4
- **Ingredients:**
  1. 1/4 cup of chia seeds
  2. 1 cup of unsweetened almond milk
  3. 1 tablespoon of honey
  4. 1/2 teaspoon of vanilla extract

5. Fresh fruit for topping

- **Instructions:**
    1. In a bowl, whisk together the chia seeds, almond milk, honey, and vanilla extract.
    2. Cover and refrigerate overnight.
    3. Stir the pudding and divide into small bowls or cups.
    4. Top with fresh fruit.
    5. Serve chilled.

6.3.3 Baked Pears with Walnuts and Honey

- **Prep Time:** 10 minutes
- **Cook Time:** 20 minutes
- **Servings:** 4
- **Ingredients:**
    1. 4 pears, halved and cored
    2. 1/4 cup of chopped walnuts
    3. 2 tablespoons of honey
    4. 1/2 teaspoon of ground cinnamon
- **Instructions:**

1. Preheat the oven to 375°F (190°C).
2. Place the pear halves in a baking dish, cut side up.
3. Sprinkle the chopped walnuts over the pears.
4. Drizzle with honey and sprinkle with ground cinnamon.
5. Bake for 20 minutes, until the pears are tender.
6. Serve warm.

These no-point dessert recipes are a great way to satisfy your sweet tooth while staying on track with your healthy eating plan. Enjoy these delicious and nutritious options guilt-free!

Chapter 7: Zero Stress Food Lists and Cooking Measurements

Eating healthy and preparing delicious meals becomes much easier when you have a well-stocked kitchen and a good understanding of basic cooking measurements. This chapter provides you with comprehensive no-point food lists, essential pantry staples, conversion charts, and tips for stress-free grocery shopping.

7.1 Comprehensive No-Point Food List

The no-point system emphasizes whole, unprocessed foods that are naturally low in calories and high in nutrients. Here is a comprehensive list of no-point foods that you can enjoy freely:

Fruits:

- Apples
- Bananas

- Berries (strawberries, blueberries, raspberries, blackberries)
- Grapes
- Oranges
- Pears
- Pineapple
- Melons (watermelon, cantaloupe, honeydew)

Vegetables:

- Leafy greens (spinach, kale, lettuce, arugula)
- Broccoli
- Cauliflower
- Carrots
- Bell peppers
- Zucchini
- Tomatoes
- Cucumbers
- Mushrooms
- Asparagus
- Green beans
- Snap peas

Proteins:

- Skinless chicken breast
- Turkey breast
- Fish (salmon, tuna, cod, tilapia)
- Shellfish (shrimp, crab, lobster)
- Eggs
- Non-fat Greek yogurt
- Cottage cheese
- Tofu
- Lentils
- Chickpeas
- Black beans
- Edamame

Grains:

- Quinoa
- Brown rice
- Oats

Others:

- Herbs and spices (basil, cilantro, parsley, thyme, rosemary, cumin, paprika)
- Garlic

- Ginger
- Lemon juice
- Lime juice
- Vinegars (apple cider vinegar, balsamic vinegar)

7.2 Pantry Staples for No-Point Cooking

Having a well-stocked pantry ensures that you always have the ingredients needed to whip up healthy and delicious no-point meals. Here are some essential pantry staples for no-point cooking:

Canned Goods:

- Canned beans (black beans, chickpeas, kidney beans)
- Canned tomatoes (diced, crushed, tomato sauce)
- Canned tuna or salmon

Grains and Pasta:

- Quinoa
- Brown rice
- Whole-grain pasta

- Rolled oats

Oils and Vinegars:

- Olive oil
- Coconut oil
- Sesame oil
- Apple cider vinegar
- Balsamic vinegar

Spices and Seasonings:

- Salt
- Black pepper
- Cumin
- Paprika
- Chili powder
- Garlic powder
- Onion powder
- Italian seasoning
- Curry powder
- Cinnamon

Condiments and Sauces:

- Soy sauce
- Hot sauce

- Mustard
- Tahini
- Nut butters (peanut butter, almond butter)

Nuts and Seeds:

- Almonds
- Walnuts
- Chia seeds
- Flax seeds
- Sunflower seeds

Baking Essentials:

- Baking powder
- Baking soda
- Vanilla extract
- Unsweetened cocoa powder
- Honey or maple syrup (for occasional use)

7.3   Conversions and Cooking Measurements

Accurate measurements are crucial for cooking success. Here are some common conversions and cooking measurements to help you in the kitchen:

Volume Conversions:

- 1 tablespoon = 3 teaspoons
- 1 cup = 16 tablespoons
- 1 pint = 2 cups
- 1 quart = 2 pints
- 1 gallon = 4 quarts

Weight Conversions:

- 1 ounce = 28 grams
- 1 pound = 16 ounces
- 1 kilogram = 2.2 pounds

Temperature Conversions:

- °F to °C: Subtract 32, then multiply by 5/9
- °C to °F: Multiply by 9/5, then add 32

Common Cooking Measurements:

- Pinch = 1/8 teaspoon
- Dash = 1/16 teaspoon
- 1 cup of flour = 120 grams
- 1 cup of sugar = 200 grams
- 1 cup of butter = 227 grams (or 2 sticks)

7.4   Tips   for   Stress-Free   Grocery Shopping

Grocery shopping can be a daunting task, but with a few tips, you can make it a stress-free and enjoyable experience:

Plan Ahead:

- Make a weekly meal plan and create a shopping list based on the recipes you plan to cook. This helps you stay organized and ensures you buy only what you need.

Stick to the Perimeter:

- The perimeter of the grocery store is where you'll find fresh produce, dairy, and meats. Focus on these sections and avoid the processed foods in the center aisles.

Shop Seasonal and Local:

- Seasonal produce is often fresher, tastier, and more affordable. Visit local farmers' markets for the best selection.

Read Labels:

- When buying packaged foods, read the labels to check for added sugars, unhealthy fats, and artificial ingredients. Choose items with simple, whole ingredients.

Don't Shop Hungry:

- Shopping on an empty stomach can lead to impulse buys and unhealthy choices. Eat a healthy snack before heading to the store.

Buy in Bulk:

- For pantry staples like grains, beans, and nuts, buying in bulk can save money and reduce packaging waste.

Use Reusable Bags:

- Bring your reusable shopping bags to reduce plastic waste and make carrying your groceries easier.

By following these tips and keeping your kitchen well-stocked with no-point foods and essential pantry staples, you can simplify your cooking routine and enjoy stress-free meal preparation. Happy cooking and shopping!

Chapter 8: Creating Your Personalized Meal Plan

Creating a personalized meal plan is key to staying on track with your no-point journey. A well-thought-out plan ensures you enjoy a variety of delicious meals while meeting your nutritional needs and weight loss goals. This chapter will guide you through the process of designing a meal plan that fits your lifestyle and keeps you motivated.

8.1 Designing Your Personalized Meal Plan

Creating a meal plan involves considering your daily schedule, dietary preferences, and nutritional requirements. Here's a step-by-step guide to help you design a personalized no-point meal plan:

Step 1: Assess Your Needs and Goals

- Determine your daily caloric needs based on your weight, height, age, gender, and activity level.

- Set specific goals for weight loss, maintenance, or muscle gain.
- Identify any dietary restrictions or preferences (e.g., vegetarian, gluten-free).

Step 2: Plan Balanced Meals

- Aim for balanced meals that include a mix of lean proteins, vegetables, fruits, whole grains, and healthy fats.
- Ensure each meal is satisfying and nutrient-dense to keep you full and energized.

Step 3: Choose a Variety of Recipes

- Select a variety of recipes from this cookbook to keep your meals interesting.
- Incorporate different cuisines and cooking methods to add diversity to your diet.

Step 4: Create a Weekly Menu

- Plan your breakfasts, lunches, dinners, and snacks for the week.
- Use a meal planning template or app to organize your menu.

Step 5: Make a Shopping List

- Based on your weekly menu, create a detailed shopping list of the ingredients you need.
- Check your pantry and fridge to see what you already have and avoid duplicates.

Step 6: Meal Prep and Cook Ahead

- Dedicate a day or two each week to meal prep. Cook and portion out meals in advance to save time during busy weekdays.
- Store prepped meals in the fridge or freezer for easy access.

Sample No-Point Weekly Meal Plan

Monday

- Breakfast: Berry Blast Smoothie
- Lunch: Mediterranean Chickpea Salad
- Dinner: Lemon Herb Grilled Chicken with steamed broccoli
- Snack: Fresh Veggie Sticks with Greek Yogurt Tzatziki

Tuesday

- Breakfast: Green Detox Smoothie
- Lunch: Asian Cabbage Salad
- Dinner: Shrimp and Vegetable Paella
- Snack: Hard-Boiled Eggs

Wednesday

- Breakfast: Peanut Butter Banana Smoothie
- Lunch: Turkey and Avocado Wrap
- Dinner: Baked Salmon with Dill and Lemon, served with quinoa
- Snack: Apple Slices with Almond Butter

Thursday

- Breakfast: Orange Creamsicle Smoothie
- Lunch: Mexican Black Bean Salad
- Dinner: Spicy Tofu Stir-Fry
- Snack: Grilled Pineapple with Lime

Friday

- Breakfast: Greek Yogurt with Berries
- Lunch: Lentil and Vegetable Stew
- Dinner: Quinoa and Black Bean Stuffed Sweet Potatoes
- Snack: Cucumber Bites with Smoked Salmon

Saturday

- Breakfast: Berry Parfait
- Lunch: Chicken and Vegetable Soup
- Dinner: Spaghetti Squash with Marinara Sauce
- Snack: Baked Zucchini Chips

Sunday

- Breakfast: Chocolate Banana Smoothie
- Lunch: Hummus and Veggie Sandwich
- Dinner: Beef and Quinoa Stuffed Peppers
- Snack: Peanut Butter Energy Balls

8.2 Staying Motivated on Your No-Point Journey

Staying motivated is crucial for long-term success on your no-point journey. Here are some strategies to help you stay committed and inspired:

Set Realistic Goals

- Set achievable short-term and long-term goals. Celebrate small victories along the way to keep yourself motivated.

Track Your Progress

- Keep a food journal or use a mobile app to track your meals, exercise, and progress. Seeing your achievements can boost your motivation.

Stay Accountable

- Share your goals with a friend or join a support group. Having someone to share your journey with can provide encouragement and accountability.

Mix It Up

- Avoid monotony by trying new recipes and experimenting with different ingredients. This keeps your meals exciting and prevents boredom.

Reward Yourself

- Treat yourself to non-food rewards for reaching milestones. Consider new workout gear, a relaxing spa day, or a fun activity you enjoy.

Stay Positive

- Focus on the positive changes you're making for your health rather than fixating on setbacks. Remember that progress takes time and persistence.

Find Inspiration

- Follow health and fitness blogs, social media accounts, or YouTube channels for inspiration and tips. Seeing others' success stories can be highly motivating.

Practice Self-Care

- Ensure you get enough sleep, manage stress, and take time for yourself. A healthy mind contributes to a healthy body and helps you stay on track.

Plan for Challenges

- Anticipate challenges such as social events, holidays, or busy schedules.

Plan ahead to make healthy choices and stay on track.

Stay Educated

- Continuously educate yourself about nutrition, healthy eating habits, and fitness. Knowledge empowers you to make informed decisions.

By following these strategies and creating a personalized meal plan, you can stay motivated and enjoy a successful no-point journey. Remember, the goal is to create a sustainable, healthy lifestyle that you enjoy and can maintain in the long run.

Conclusion

Recap of Key Takeaways

Throughout this book, we've explored how to make healthy eating enjoyable and stress-free with no-point recipes. Here are the key takeaways from each chapter:

Chapter 1: Energizing Breakfasts

- Start your day with nutritious, no-point breakfasts to keep you energized and satisfied.
- Quick and easy breakfast ideas, high-protein options, smoothies, and overnight oats are great choices.

Chapter 2: Satisfying Lunches

- Enjoy balanced, no-point lunches with salads, soups, wraps, and meal prep tips.
- Incorporate a variety of flavors and ingredients to keep your meals interesting and nutritious.

Chapter 3: Delicious Dinners

- Create satisfying and healthy dinners with one-pot meals, flavorful main courses, vegetarian and vegan options, and family-friendly recipes.
- Focus on lean proteins, vegetables, and whole grains for balanced meals.

Chapter 4: Snacks and Appetizers

- Choose no-point snacks and appetizers that are quick, healthy, and satisfying.
- Options include fresh veggie sticks, dips, guilt-free appetizers, and crunchy snacks.

Chapter 5: Smoothies

- Smoothies are a convenient and nutritious option for any time of the day.
- Use a variety of fruits, vegetables, and protein sources to create refreshing no-point smoothies.

Chapter 6: Desserts

- Indulge in no-point desserts that are both delicious and healthy.
- Enjoy fruit-based desserts, no-bake treats, and indulgent yet nutritious options.

Chapter 7: Zero Stress Food Lists and Cooking Measurements

- Stock your pantry with essential no-point foods and ingredients.
- Use cooking measurement conversions and stress-free grocery shopping tips to simplify your meal preparation.

Chapter 8: Creating Your Personalized Meal Plan

- Design a personalized meal plan that fits your lifestyle and dietary needs.
- Stay motivated with realistic goals, tracking progress, and finding inspiration.

Final Thoughts and Encouragement

Embarking on a no-point journey is about more than just losing weight; it's about adopting a healthier lifestyle that you can sustain long-term. By incorporating the recipes and tips in this book, you can enjoy delicious meals without the stress of counting points or calories. Remember, the key to success is consistency and enjoying the process. Celebrate your progress, stay positive, and keep experimenting with new recipes and flavors. Your journey to better health is a lifelong adventure—embrace it with enthusiasm and curiosity.

Acknowledgements

I would like to express my gratitude to everyone who has supported me in creating this book. Special thanks to my family and friends for their encouragement and feedback throughout the writing process. I also want to thank the readers for choosing this book and trusting me to guide them on their journey to healthier eating.